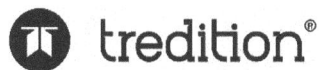

D1785455

Samesh Ramjattan

Fix Your Depression & Anxiety

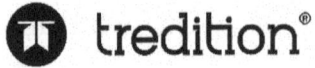

Copyright © 2018 Samesh Ramjattan

Publisher: tredition, Hamburg, Germany

ISBN
Paperback: 978-3-7439-9441-6
eBook: 978-3-7439-9443-0

Printed on demand in many countries

All rights reserved. No part of this publication may be reproduced, distributed, or transmitted in any form or by any means, including photocopying, recording, or other electronic or mechanical methods, without the prior written permission of the publisher, except in the case of brief quotations embodied in critical reviews and certain other noncommercial uses permitted by copyright law. For permission requests, write to the publish

LET THE HEALING BEGIN

You have a higher purpose. You've always felt it and yet somehow you have chosen to ignore it and settle for a life that is routed in a much lower state and vibration. In order to maintain this lower state, you have sought out stimulation in the form of a daily fix of subscription to social media, movies, television, music, fast food, sex, drugs and alcohol. You imagine yourself as an icon, predefined by the rest of the world - others like you, who seem to be addicted to the same things. It's a vicious, cruel and brazen world where no prisoners are taken, and those that cannot conform wither into an unrecognised, unreported and weaker sub world that nobody cares to acknowledge, all because nobody wants to admit that they are secretly members too.

But this world and its citizenship grows by the day, filling with new arrivals who have fallen from the supposed glossy surface with its manufactured personas that only illustrate flawless complexions, rose-tinted eyes, perfectly tanned lean bodies, vivacious personalities, flowing champagne, fast cars, unlimited cash and consequence free sex. This world has no time for old fashioned values, traditions, emotions, loyalty, love or meaning. It is disposable, a fleeting impression worth only the three-second 'view' or 'like'. Maintaining this elaborate production is exhausting, draining of your precious Self, identity and individuality, like featuring in a 24-7 Big Brother style reality TV show of you own life. And that's when things begin to flounder. All is not well. Maintaining this contrived persona becomes too much for a delicate constitution that was never designed for this. Like an overworked machine – no longer able to prop up a perpetual, everlasting charade - it fails. Running on empty - energy, mood and life force goes into low ebb. Low emotions prompt feelings of dread, despair and worthlessness and a tendency to cry at any moment, feeling like you are living under a grey cloud. Low vibration and energy leaves you unable to face the frenetic world during the day, but as the world quietens into slumber, you feel unusually revitalised, seeking to recharge by opting for stimulants such as drugs, alcohol, fast food and sugar, providing the fix you need to once again join the nation of stimulation. But while the rest of the world, who can by some limited measure keep their subscription to mesmerisation under control, sleep, you toil in the Twittersphere, blatantly denying your condition and only serving to further exacerbate it. Again, when this fire burns itself out and the fuel is exhausted, you crash and burn, useless to everything and everyone around you, especially yourself.

While I give you some empathy, for I myself have been there, YOU are the one who got yourself to this place. And only YOU can get yourself out. Modern medicine calls this affliction Depression and Anxiety, but we should call it what it really is – an addiction to stimulation. You are a Stimulation Mutation, and the only way to fix yourself is to cut off the drug at the supply. In this short book, I will provide you with 3 simple ways to fix this condition. It is simple, free, drug-free, and can be practised by anybody, anywhere. All you need is your own commitment, and you can return to health, well-being and happiness. You *can* choose you own destiny and in turn you can overcome anything if you just present enough will to do. Think about it. The amount of will each of us dedicates to being famous, popular, successful and wealthy, can easily be diverted toward creating change in our lives, even if it is just a little bit. Now that change will involve discipline and dedication. All I can say is – its up to you. If you are reading this then you probably sought out change in the first place, and knowledge finds those who truly seek it.

Now I know what you are going to say – that this is fault of the world. The media, social and otherwise, technology, convenience (beauty, food, drugs and alcohol), and so on, but as the parade went passed, you chose to cheer and then you didn't stop there – you wanted to be a part of that parade, wanting to experience the jubilation every day and then every minute. Now you can't do without it and you've invented a 'persona', an unhealthy illusion of your true self that cannot be perpetually maintained and now you find yourself in a very deep, dark hole, hoping that somebody will just throw you a lifeline. And many have probably tried – family, friends, medical professionals. But the hardest part is that you feel like nobody understands or identifies with your predicament, because they can't see how hard it is to be in this deep, dark hole, and you are fed-up of being down there at the bottom – cold and alone. Well in this book, I am going to jump in there with you, and your response might be; "Are you crazy? Now we are both stuck down here in this hole."

But the difference is, is that I know how to get out, and I am going to show you how too.

The reality is that each and everyone has suffered from depression at some point in their lives. They are just capable of hiding it very well. Many have chosen not to speak of it for fear of ridicule or lack of empathy. Many still do suffer from it and will continue to bounce in and out of it depending on the particular circumstances in their lives. In the past, the affliction was misunderstood and misdiagnosed, with medical professionals baffled by it and unsure how to treat it. Indeed, much of this misunderstanding still exists, and the quick-fix seems to favour prescription of antidepressants. But often, recipients of this treatment, claim to not be themselves or are unable to live a normal life whilst on these drugs. Some also experience side-effects and for some the drugs simply do not work at all, leaving them worse off. If it is your intention not to resort to drugs and you would like to opt for a more holistic, spiritual approach that can heal you and further enhance your life, then read on and practise these simple techniques.

BALANCING THE EGO

In my book, BE YOUR HIGHER SELF, I go in to great discussion about the Ego, but for the purposes of this novella, I will briefly introduce it as it is vital in understanding it so that you may be able to counter its influence. Firstly, what is the ego? I am sure you have heard of it time and time again, banded about by psychiatrists and psychologists. Quite simply, the ego is the conscious mind, which provides us with our sense of identity and an inflated feeling of pride in feeling superior to others. And it is this mechanism in our central programming that makes us see ourselves as individuals striving for prolonged self-determination. In other words, as long as I am better off than others, I am better off by myself.

There are principally only two major emotions – Love and Fear.

All positive emotions come from love, all negative emotions from fear. From love flows happiness, contentment, peace and joy. From fear comes anger, hate, anxiety and guilt. The ego resides in the part of the body related to lower vibration and energy, and propagates the emotions of fear, that fuel depression and anxiety. Often the low vibration of the ego ends up overstimulated, and fears such as failure, survival, rejection, inadequacy, intimacy, unpredictability, uncertainty and death create symptoms of anxiety, loneliness, anger, hatred, isolation, stress and physical symptoms such as illness and disease.

The world now celebrates this permanent state of repression as normal, defining this current state as our reality; however, it is down to each of us to balance our egos, re-establish the connection to our higher selves, and by doing so change our existence.

To better understand how the effects on the ego, we must also explore the masculine and feminine energies that co-exist within us.

We are all born male or female, but we are not born masculine or feminine. We all have both masculine and feminine energies within us, yet we may not be fully aware of what these look like, or that they even exist. Furthermore, most of us are content to believe that these energies simply define our behaviour in the form of gender alone.

Masculine energy is independent and analytical, representing our left brain and body. When it is used properly, it is assertive, practical and visionary. When masculine energy is unbalanced and dominates our existence, it draws on the ego, perpetuating anger, resentment and inner conflict that disconnect our higher selves from our bodies, inhibiting the flow of energy between the body's energy points or chakras. The masculine is a necessary trait, for it supports the growth of a balanced ego, financial stability, family, shelter and organisation.

Feminine energy is an intelligent and loving energy that contains the quality of our intuition, compassion, emotion, empathy and truth. When you are strong in your feminine, you have a strong connection to your body, intuition, receptivity, dreams and emotions. It is a necessary counterbalance to the masculine, and you can make decisions based on what you feel in your heart. Feminine energy is a creative, right-brain and body energy. Yet, if we are too much in our feminine, we can come across as weak and lose our personal sense of power.

Both energies are vital for effective existence; however, if these energies are unbalanced, they promote discord, unhappiness and illness. A practice that we will explore later is Alternate nostril breathing. This is an uplifting and calming breathing practice that works directly with the right and left sides of the body and brain to cultivate harmony and mental clarity, promoting energy flows that help clear blocked energy streams in the body and establish a reconnection with the higher self.

You need to understand that having an energetic balance brings wholeness, softness and strength which will rebalance the ego with the higher self, and fix the symptoms of depression and anxiety, as well as other mental and physical illnesses.

STEP 1 - MEDITATION

Now you may think that meditation is for 'flakes' or is a bunch of 'hocus pocus', but as I mentioned earlier, perhaps it is time to alter your perception and belief systems of what you think is your true reality. The journey of a thousand steps begins with a single one, so its up to you whether you wish to take it or not. Remember, you are the one at the bottom of a hole, and this is the way out.

ALTERNATE NOSTRIL BREATHING:

Alternate nostril breathing is a simple yet powerful and effective technique that settles the mind, body and emotions. You can use it to quieten your mind before beginning a meditation practice; and it is particularly helpful to ease racing thoughts if you are experiencing depression, anxiety, stress or having trouble sleeping.

With just a few minutes of alternate nostril breathing, you can energetically realign the mind and body, and restore necessary balance.

In addition to calming the mind and reversing stress, alternate nostril breathing also improves our ability to focus the mind, supports lung and respiratory functions which boost the immune system, rejuvenates the nervous system and removes toxins. However, the vital benefit is to restore balance in the masculine and feminine energies and balance the ego that gives rise to the anxiety and stress in the first place.

Alternate nostril breathing is a quick and calming way to bring you back to your centre, particularly if you find it difficult to settle into your meditations.

1.   Find a quiet room that is well lit and well ventilated.

2.   Sit in a comfortable seat, making sure your spine is straight and your heart is open.

3.   Relax your left palm comfortably into your lap and bring your right hand just in front of your face.

4.   With your right hand, bring your index finger and middle finger together to rest between your eyebrows, lightly using them as an anchor. The fingers we will be actively using are the thumb and ring finger.

5.   Close your eyes and take a deep breath in and out through your nose.

6.   Close your right nostril with your right thumb. Inhale through the left nostril slowly and steadily.

7.   Close the left nostril with your ring finger so both nostrils are held closed; retain your breath at the top of the inhale for a brief pause.

8.   Open your right nostril and release the breath slowly through the right side; pause briefly at the bottom of the exhale.

9.   Inhale through the right side slowly.

10. Hold both nostrils closed (with ring finger and thumb).

11. Open your left nostril and release breath slowly through the left side. Pause briefly at the bottom.

12. Repeat for nine cycles, or about five minutes, allowing your mind to follow your inhales and exhales. Your exhalation should be longer than your inhalation.

13. Steps 6-11 represent one complete cycle of alternate nostril breathing. If you're moving through the sequence slowly, one cycle should take you about thirty-forty seconds. Move through nine cycles when you're feeling stressed, anxious or in need of a rebalance.

High frequency vibration and the energy of love will help to combat the ego-driven lower vibration-induced emotions linked to fear. Without the neces-sary tools and aids, this is no simple task, especially in a world where the fuel for such ego stimulation is so readily available, almost everywhere we turn. The first of these tools are mantras and their use with meditation.

Mantras are powerful Sanskrit words, whose sounds or utterances, when repeated in succession, have the power to balance lower vibrational energy throughout the chakras and reconnect with the hig-her self and cosmic energy. Mantras form the basis of all religious traditions, scriptures and prayers and can help alter your ego-fuelled impulses, habits and afflictions. Mantras are meant to bring you back to the path of health, well-being and happiness.

I have chosen two specific mantras to use with meditating, helping you on your road to recovery:

Om Ram Ramaya Namaha

(OM RAHM RAHM-EE-YAH NAHM-AH-HA)

This is a very powerful traditional Sanskrit mantra, that can cure many ills including depression and anxiety.

However, if you are uncomfortable with, or have difficulty using this mantra, then you can also use the following:

Every day in every way, I'm getting better and better

PRACTISING MEDITATION:

- Choose a peaceful environment

Meditation should be practised in a peaceful, tranquil environment which will enable you to focus and avoid external stimuli and distractions. Find a place where you will not be interrupted for the duration of your meditation, whether it lasts five minutes or half an hour. The space does not need to be very large – a walk-in closet or even an outdoor bench can be used for meditation as long as you have privacy and are without any external distractions such as TVs, radios, phones or other noisy appliances.

Your meditation space does not need to be completely silent, so you won't need earplugs. The sound of a lawnmower or dog barking shouldn't prevent effective meditation. In fact, being aware of the noises of your natural environment without letting them dominate your thoughts is an important component of meditation. However, avoid a busy roadway or other sources of loud noise. Finding peace under a tree or sitting upon some lush grass in a favourite corner of a garden would be ideal.

- Decide on the length of your meditation

Before you begin, you should decide how long you are going to meditate. While many seasoned meditators recommend twenty-minute sessions twice a day, you can start by doing as little as five minutes once a day, especially if you cannot initially find the time. But you will be surprised how you will find the time should you intend to. You should also try to meditate at the same time each day, whether it's fifteen minutes first thing in the morning or five minutes on your lunch hour. Whatever length of time you choose, try to make meditation a regular part of your daily routine. Do not feel embarrassment in informing your family, partners or work colleagues that you need to take time to meditate. You will be amazed how considerate people can be.

Once you have decided on a time frame, try to stick to it. Don't just give up because you feel like it isn't working, as it will take time and regular practice to achieve successful meditation. Initially, the most important thing is to persist.

Find a way to keep track of your meditation time without distracting yourself. Set a gentle alarm to alert you when your time is up or keep a slight eye on the time on a watch or wall clock.

- Sit in a comfortable position

It is very important that you are comfortable while you meditate, so finding the best position for you is key. Traditionally, meditation is practised by sitting on a cushion on the ground in either a lotus position or half-lotus position, but this position can be uncomfortable if you lack flexibility in your legs, hips and lower back. You want to find a posture that works for you.

You can sit in a chair or sofa, ensuring that you are comfortable, relaxed, and have a balanced torso, so your spine can support all your weight from the waist up, while resting your hands on your knees or leaving them hanging down by your side.

- Close your eyes

Meditation can be performed with the eyes open or closed; however, it is best to try meditating with closed eyes to avoid visual distractions.

Don't worry if your mind starts to wander. Just try to refocus your mind on your breathing and try to think of nothing else.

- Repeat the mantra

Mantra meditation involves repeating a mantra over and over, creating vibrations in the mind, allowing you to disconnect from your thoughts and enter a deeper state of consciousness, connecting your higher self and your chakras.

Silently repeat the mantra over and over to yourself as you meditate, allowing the word or phrase to echo through your mind. Don't worry if your mind wanders. Just refocus your attention and on the repetition of the word.

As you enter a deeper level of awareness and consciousness, it may become unnecessary to continue repeating the mantra. Daily meditation will produce more profound benefits, especially early morning as your mind has not yet become consumed with the stresses and worries of the day.

However, do not meditate directly after eating as you may feel uncomfortable and less able to concentrate if you're digesting a meal. It is perfectly natural for the mind to wander and pay attention to the images and messages that appear during meditation, especially as you become more experienced.

Many of the impressions experienced during meditation are powerful messages regarding karma and aspects of the ego that are released, as the higher vibrations liberate negative energies from the chakras via the higher self connection. Allow these to appear and resolve naturally, bearing in mind that anything of importance will be retained after meditation. It is important to pay attention to these insights and note them down in a spiritual journal.

STEP 2 - YOU ARE WHAT YOU EAT

I am sure you are questioning the reasoning behind including a chapter on diet and nutrition in a book about dealing with depression and anxiety. However, these days no spiritual transformation could be attempted without priming the body with higher vibration cleansing; and that begins with what you put into it. Indeed, there is a causal relationship between the higher self and the compulsions of lower self, most notably what we feed ourselves.

Food in these modern times has become the convenient and abundant 'fix', fuelling an addiction which is escaping our need to survive and evolving into a leisurely obsession of feeding our faces toward a permanent gluttonous, unhealthy epidemic. Food and drink manufacturers continue to think up more inventive and innovative ways to feed our hunger for convenience, speed and value. Resistance is indeed futile; however, there is hope, and resistance comes in the form of rehabilitation from the drug that holds us in its grip.

- Detoxification

The body retains fat as protection against the overproduction of acids produced by a typical unhealthy modern diet, causing a congested bowel and sluggish digestion that can both increase the fat load in the body.

The body is naturally primed to combat normal amounts of toxins; however, abnormally high levels of toxins through consumption of sugar, processed foods, alcohol and high levels of saturated fat can affect your metabolic rate, digestion and the production of fat. By removing the foods that are high in such toxins and consuming foods that help the body detox, the body becomes more alkaline, or less acidic, so the fat is no longer needed, increasing your metabolic rate and therefore helping you burn fat faster.

The effects of a 'detox' go far beyond being just a physical cleanse or a good way to lose excess weight; it is a powerful way to balance and re-energise the chakras. When you make a change in your physical body you will see that change joyfully expressed in your wellbeing too.

Your body can accumulate toxins for many years without any recourse, but eventually when your organs and vital systems can no longer cope, the body starts to resist, and at this point of personal excess you will experience disease. These toxins have a direct effect on the function of the chakras, causing them to become over or underactive, or blocked altogether. These may start out as frequent ailments such as coughs and colds or regular headaches and, if left unaided, develop into obesity, high blood pressure, high cholesterol, arthritis or diabetes to name but a few.

The process of effective fasting and detoxification helps to release and eliminate unwanted toxins in a safe way, supporting the body's ability to heal itself, by energising and balancing chakras and eliminating health issues.

Some of the benefits of a detox are greater vitality and more consistent energy, improved digestion and absorption of nutrients; improved fertility; relief from chronic health problems such as skin conditions, including eczema, psoriasis and acne; Irritable Bowel Syndrome (IBS); migraines; improved hormonal balance; weight loss and enhanced metabolic function; strengthened immune system and greater emotional and mental well-being.

- Detox Plan

Committing to any detox plan can be difficult, as it will require a great deal of dedication and discipline. However, at the end of it you will wonder how you ever allowed things to get so bad, as the compulsions and cravings disappear, the mental fog lifts and you begin to feel revitalised.

Detox plans can run from seven to twenty-one days in succession, depending on how severe the effects or symptoms of ill health are. I would recommend a seven-day plan and take stock of how you feel. Then perhaps recommence the regime a few days or weeks thereafter.

Plan the timing of your detox effectively, as you will be required to plan and prepare your meals over the period, and it is pointless to coincide the detox with a busy week at work or during the kids' summer holidays. A great deal of fortitude and willpower will be required, so prepare yourself as if you were preparing for a marathon. Think of it as checking yourself into rehab. Believe me, in the first few days it will feel like that, as you attempt to wean yourself off the toxic addiction, but it will be worth it in the end. During the initial stages of the detox you will experience headaches, bloating and increased bowel and bladder movements as the body begins to rebalance and expel toxins. However, as you progress you will begin to feel better, lighter and more coherent. You will no longer crave toxic foods, and a euphoric state will begin to prevail. During this period, intensify your meditations and ensure you practise the alternate nostril breathing.

Drink at least two litres of water per day and get plenty of sleep – at least eight hours a night.

- Foods to include in the plan:

- Dairy substitutes: Rice and nut milks such as almond milk and coconut milk
- Non-gluten grains: brown rice, millet, amaranth, teff, tapioca, buckwheat, potato flour, quinoa and gluten-free oats
- Fruits and vegetables: unsweetened fresh or frozen whole fruits, diluted fruit juices and raw, steamed, sautéed, juiced or roasted vegetables

- Animal protein: fresh or water-packed fish, wild game, lamb, duck, organic chicken and turkey
- Vegetable protein: split peas, lentils and legumes
- Nuts and seeds: walnuts, sesame, pumpkin and sunflower seeds, hazelnuts, pecans, almonds, cashews, nut butters such as almond or tahini
- Oils: cold-pressed olive, flax, safflower, sesame, almond, sunflower, walnut, canola and pumpkin
- Drinks: filtered or distilled water, decaffeinated herbal teas, sparkling or still mineral water
- Sweeteners: brown rice syrup, agave nectar, stevia, fruit sweetener and blackstrap molasses
- Condiments: vinegar; all spices, including salt, pepper, basil, carob, cinnamon, cumin, dill, garlic, ginger, mustard, oregano, parsley, rosemary, tarragon, thyme and turmeric

- Foods to exclude from your plan:

- All dairy and eggs
- All butter and mayonnaise
- Grains: wheat, corn, barley, spelt, rye, most oats (oats are usually contaminated with gluten unless you can find a gluten-free brand)
- Fruits and vegetables: oranges, orange juice, corn, creamed vegetables, canned fruit and vegetables

- Animal protein: pork, beef, veal, sausage, cold cuts, canned meats, frankfurters, shellfish
- Vegetable protein: soybean products (soy sauce, soybean oil in processed foods such as: tempeh, tofu, soy milk, soy yogurt, textured vegetable protein)
- Nuts and seeds: peanuts and peanut butter
- Oils: shortening, processed oils, salad dressings and spreads
- Drinks: alcohol, caffeinated beverages and soft drinks
- Sweeteners: white and brown refined sugars, honey, maple syrup, high-fructose corn syrup and evaporated cane juice
- Condiments: chocolate, ketchup, relish, chutney, barbecue sauce, teriyaki

- Going Vegetarian or Vegan for a day

Once you have completed your detox, it is down to you whether you wish to continue on a longer programme. You will hopefully feel invigorated, and the need to return to the type of eating habits that brought you to this point will have changed. Personally, I like to detox every two to three months depending on how I feel. Your body will begin to provide the appropriate signals accordingly. It might also be a good idea to go vegetarian or even vegan for a day or two every week. Monday is always a good day, especially after the excesses of the weekend. This will give your body the opportunity to rebalance and expel any toxins. During these days of 'fasting', remember to consume pure, fresh and simple foods, avoiding the foods from the exclusion list above.

STEP 3 - LOVE YOURSELF

We spend our entire lives giving energy and love to others in an effort to please, because of feelings of obligation and guilt. You owe the people around nothing and you cannot spend your life, living it simply to please others, particularly their impression of what it should be. Parents, partners, friends, family and even strangers in the workplace or in society at large, have placed an invisible yoke around your neck that keeps you in a perpetual prison of expectation. We are all taught as children from an early age to be good little boys and girls, good citizens, good consumers, good patrons, good workers, good husbands and wives, and good people – spending our lives in an enslaved pre-programmed delusion, where any focus solely on ourselves is to be denied and labelled as selfish or self-centred. Now, I am not suggesting that we suddenly become selfish, self-absorbed individuals, hell bent on ignoring or treating others poorly. No. I am asserting that selflessness and charity begin at home and all self awareness begins with an introspective on who you really are. Often the behaviours and character that we exhibit in adulthood is the product of the environment which we grew up in, and while we all have a choice to forge our journeys and destinies, most of us simply give in and assimilate what is around us. We then carry these 'burdens' or fears with us and are incapable of seeking or living with love in its purity, because we are saddled with the ego-driven fears that we have harnessed since childhood. These seem to become more prolific as we age, manifesting into mental illnesses such as depression and anxiety.

So much of the fear and anxiety we harbour is a result of the poor level of self worth or love that we hold for ourselves. How often have you stood in front of the mirror and been disgusted with the image that presents back at you, even though this is just naturally who you are, and not the fake air-brushed model from the pages of a magazine? Have you studied a vocation or taken a job or career path because it is what your parents, family or culture determines? How often have you put the needs of others first, and your own last, as you tirelessly give without regard or recognition? How many times have you wished you were doing something else or, were with someone else, but stayed where you were because that was what was expected of you? How often have you felt obliged to be busy or pre-occupied rather than giving yourself time to rest or just sit by yourself?

If each of us serves what was truly in our hearts without the recourse of fears such as guilt, failure or obligation, then happiness, well-being and love would prevail, however we continue to live under the spectre of denial and delusion, while everyone around you, apart from you, benefits from your subservient enslavement.

Fixing your depression and anxiety means having the courage to confess to your inadequacies and be true to your higher self and its higher energies. Facing these fears means recovery, and this may mean making radical changes to your life such as changing your career, location, relationships and how you personally look at things. And once you 'wake' to the falsehood of your own illusion, things will seem very different, and what you perceived as truth quickly unravels into lies. But don't be afraid of this. You are setting yourself free, and by doing so – healing.

Ultimately, *You Get What You Give.* So, opportunities to change will present themselves because that is what you want deep down. You want to break free from the modern-day enslavement to overstimulation, hence you have attracted an illness that presents the opportunity to break free.

We live in a world where being alone is labelled as lonely but is truly where the elixir of truth lies. You can't find your true voice in the noise of others. The energy of healing lies in that true voice which will be discovered once the low vibrational noise of the ego is turned down, and there is no way to discover it whilst others are so fervently subscribed to that noise.

Remember to do the following to aid your healing:

- Take time out for yourself, and this may include sitting quietly either for rest or meditation, without the interruption of television, your smartphone or any other device.
- Take long walks through places with plenty of trees and nature, away from busy urban areas and shopping malls.
- Spend time in or near water, such as lakes, sea sides or rivers. Swim if can as water has remarkable high vibrational healing properties, but not in public swimming pools.
- Spend time in the company of pets and animals as they will give you unconditional love.

- Remove the toxic elements of your life! Only you will know what this means and how far you will have to go. Frequent meditation will begin to highlight certain negative emotions and energies as they rise to the surface, so don't be surprised by changes in your behaviour, especially a new-found assertiveness and forthrightness.

- Expand you spiritual awakening by reading books on the subjects that might have intrigued you from this novella. Join a meditation group, Yoga class or take Reiki treatments.

- Be prepared to let people go. Depending on where you are in your life, you may find that you must accept that it is time to move on and exclude certain people who consistently reinforce your negative feelings and actions, contributing to your condition. This might even mean people who have been close to you and have served you, but unfortunately as you leave those low vibrational fears behind, you cannot remain in a relationship with them, especially if they cannot, and are ultimately responsible for your downfall.

Turning your attention and energy to yourself will set you on the path to certain recovery, unearthing certain radical truths and even a new path for your self-discovery. Remember to embrace them with love, compassion, patience and an open mind. You have been quietly constructing your ego for a lifetime, so balancing it and bringing it under control takes time so persevere and don't give up. You are already on your way!

ALSO

BY

SAMESH RAMJATTAN

BE YOUR

HIGHER SELF

EVERYTHING YOU NEED TO KNOW TO
SIMPLY NEED TO FIX YOURSELF, ALL IN ONE
PLACE

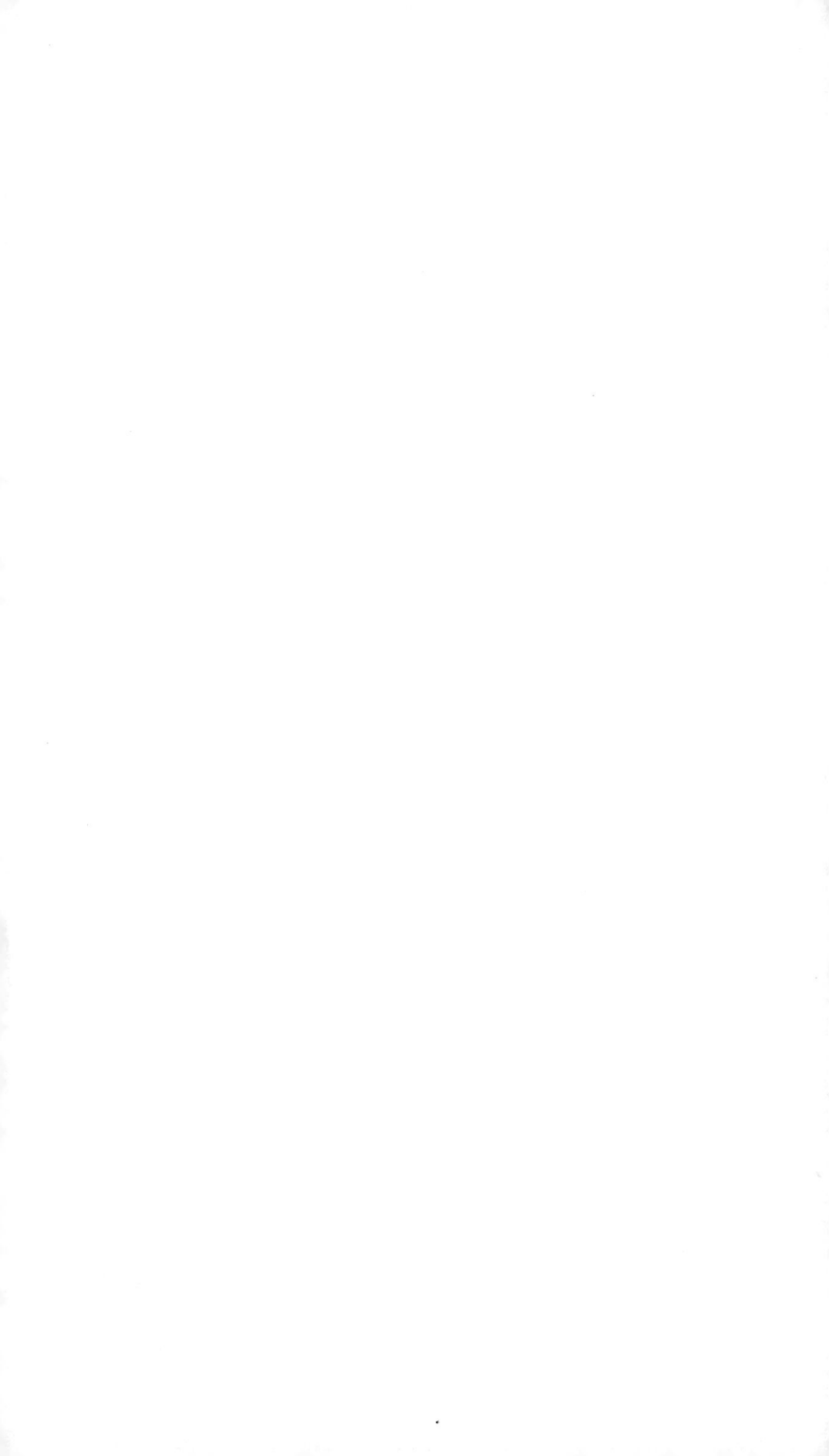

Lightning Source UK Ltd.
Milton Keynes UK
UKHW02f1551120818
327112UK00008B/396/P